Ketamine Journal

EMBRACE THE ADVENTURE:
KEEP TRACK OF YOUR PSYCHEDELIC THERAPY

Ashley Terwilliger

THANKS SO MUCH FOR BUYING MY JOURNAL! BE SURE
TO TAKE A LOOK AT MY OTHER JOURNALS AND FOLLOW
ME ON AMAZON TO STAY UPDATED ON NEW RELEASES.
YOUR SUPPORT MEANS A LOT TO ME! YOU CAN FIND
MORE OF MY WORK AT:
AMAZON.COM/AUTHOR/ASHLEYS_WRITING_CREATIONS

This Journal Belongs to:

———————————

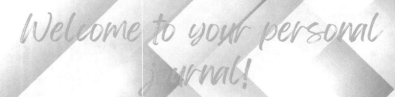

Welcome to your personal journal!

THIS SPACE IS DEDICATED TO YOUR JOURNEY THROUGH KETAMINE TREATMENT. USE THESE PROMPTS TO REFLECT ON YOUR EXPERIENCES, EMOTIONS, AND PROGRESS. YOUR THOUGHTS AND INSIGHTS ARE VALUABLE.

WRITE FREELY AND HONESTLY. THERE ARE NO RIGHT OR WRONG ANSWERS.

Preparation for Treatment:

(THESE ARE THINGS THAT I HAVE FOUND HELPFUL DURING TREATMENT DAYS)

- **MEDITATE!!! ALWAYS TRY TO GO INTO TREATMENT RELAXED & CALM. THIS MAY MAKE OR BREAK YOUR TREATMENT EXPERIENCE.**
- **STAY HYDRATED & BRING WATER WITH YOU**
- **DO NOT EAT WITHIN 1-HOUR OF YOUR APPOINTMENT IN CASE YOU GET NAUSEOUS**
- **NO CAFFEINE 6 HOURS BEFORE TREATMENT**
- **NO DRUGS OR ALCOHOL THE DAY OF TREATMENT**
- **WEAR COMFY CLOTHES. SUCH AS SWEATSHIRT, SWEATPANTS, YOGA OR WORKOUT CLOTHING. I PERSONALLY WEAR A SWEATSHIRT WITH OVERSIZE HOOD TO PULL DOWN OVER MY FACE**
- **BRING A BLANKET IF YOU TEND TO GET COLD**
- **USE NOISE CANCELLING EARBUD OR HEADPHONES SO YOU CAN FOCUS ON THE MUSIC INSTEAD OF THE SURROUNDING NOISES**
- **MAKE A PLAYLIST THAT IS AT LEAST 1-HOUR LONG OF WHATEVER TYPE OF MUSIC YOU ENJOY**

Things to Avoid After Treatment:

- **DO NOT TAKE WHAT YOU JUST EXPERIENCE LITERALLY. KETAMINE TREATMENTS TEND TO BE ABSTRACT AND DREAM LIKE.**
- **DO NOT MAKE ANY DRAMATIC CHANGES OR LARGE PURCHASES IMMEDIATELY AFTER. URGES TO MAKE CHANGES ARE COMMON AFTER TREATMENT.**
- **DO NOT OVER-STIMULATION YOURSELF, RESTING IMMEDIATELY AFTER IS RECOMMENDED**

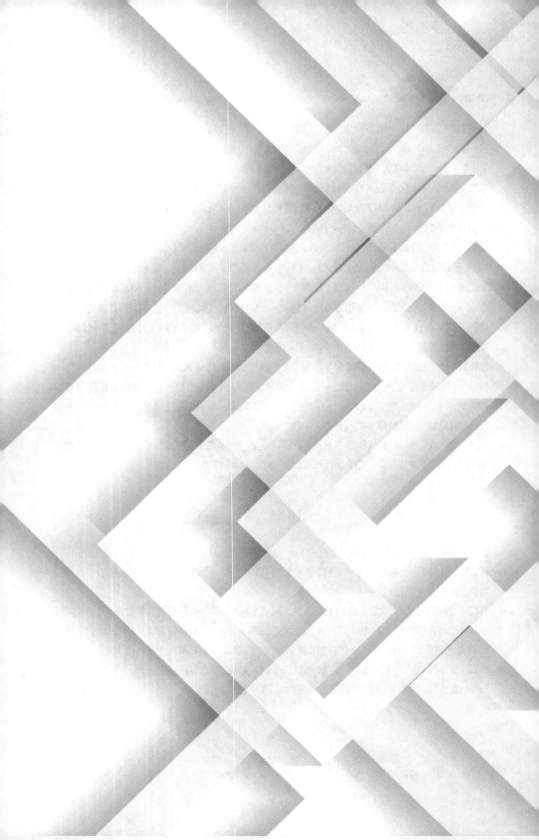

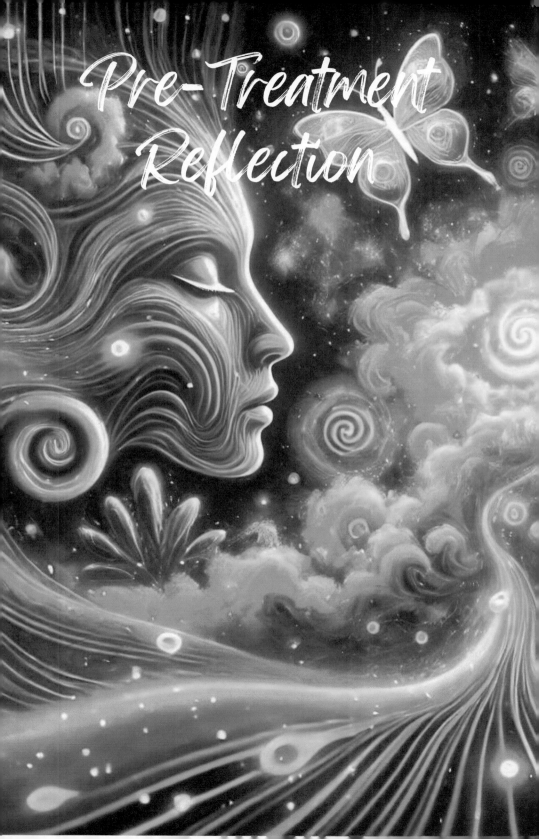

Pre-Treatment
Reflection

HOW DO YOU FEEL ABOUT STARTING KETAMINE TREATMENT?

WHAT ARE YOUR HOPES AND CONCERNS ABOUT TREATMENT?

WHAT DO YOU EXPECT TO ACHIEVE THROUGH THIS TREATMENT?

Current State of Mind

DESCRIBE YOUR CURRENT EMOTIONAL STATE

WHAT EMOTIONS ARE MOST PROMINENT FOR YOU RIGHT NOW?

WHAT HAS LED YOU TO SEEK KETAMINE TREATMENT AT THIS POINT IN YOUR LIFE?

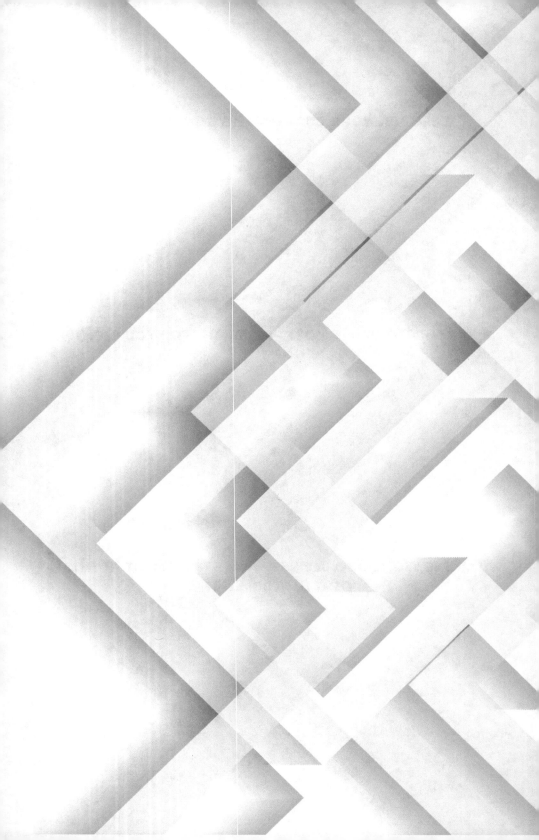

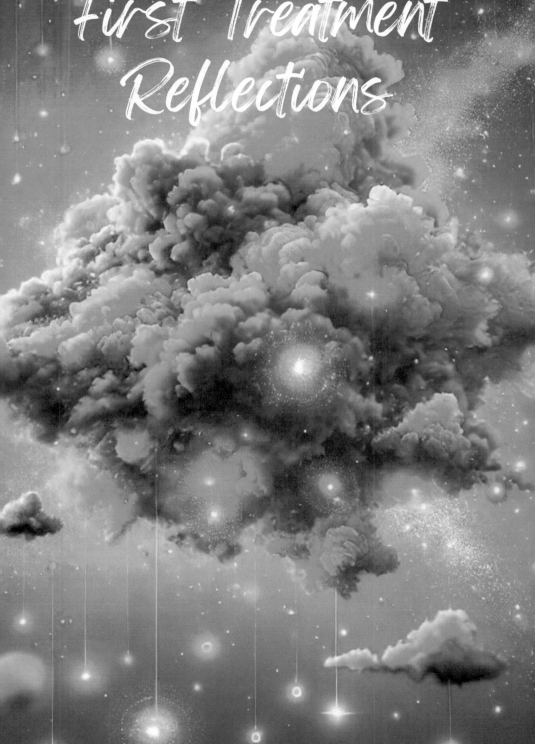

First Treatment
Reflections

First Session Experience

DESCRIBE YOUR FIRST KETAMINE TREATMENT SESSION

**WHAT WERE YOUR INITIAL REACTIONS AND FEELINGS
DURING AND AFTER THE SESSION?**

DID ANYTHING UNEXPECTED HAPPEN DURING THE SESSION?

HOW DID YOU RESPOND TO IT?

HOW DO YOU FEEL YOUR TREATMENT WENT?

DID YOU HAVE ANY PHYSICAL RESPONSES TO TREATMENT?

DO YOU THINK YOU WILL CONTINUE TREATMENT? WHY?

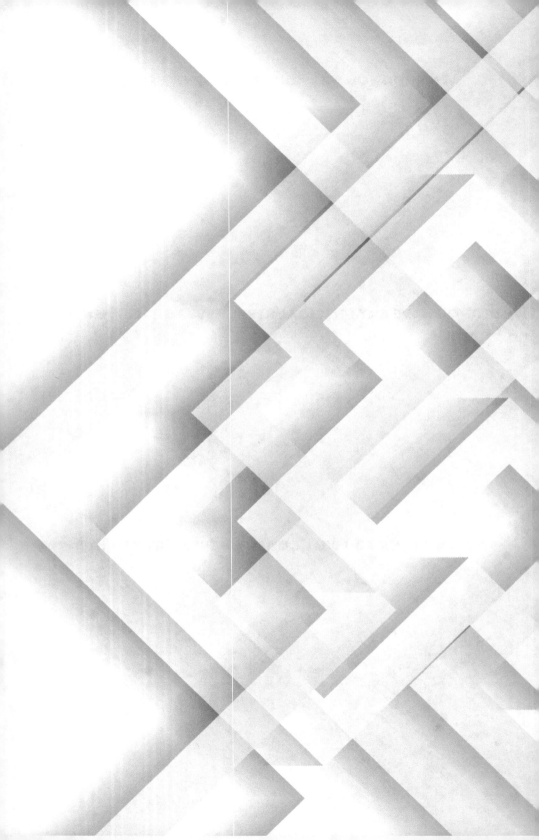

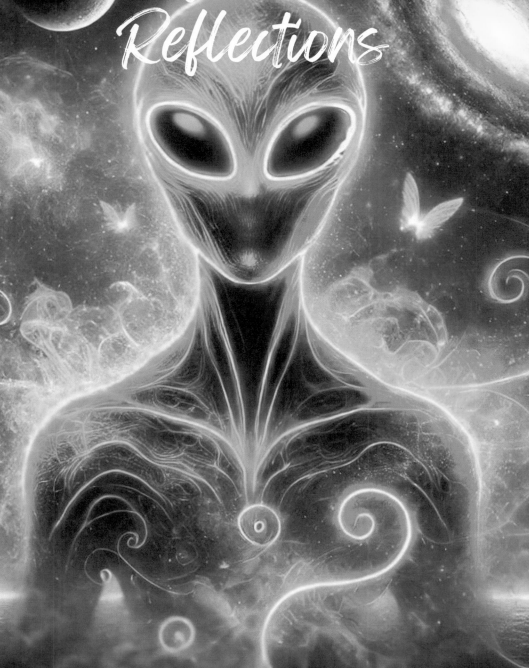

During Treatment Reflections

DATE: _____

KETAMINE DOSE: _____

WHAT IS YOUR MOOD GOING INTO THE TREATMENT?

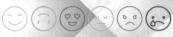

WHAT DID YOU EXPERIENCE DURING TREATMENT?

WHAT PHYSICAL SENSATIONS DID YOU NOTICE DURING YOUR TREATMENT? HOW DID THEY AFFECT YOU?

WHAT EMOTIONS SURFACED DURING THE SESSION? WERE THEY FAMILIAR OR NEW?

DID YOU EXPERIENCE ANY VISUAL CHANGES OR IMAGERY? DESCRIBE THEM IN DETAIL:

WHAT THOUGHTS OR MEMORIES CAME UP DURING YOUR TREATMENT? HOW DID YOU FEEL ABOUT THEM?

Post-Session Reflection

DID YOU DISASSOCIATE?   ◯**YES**   ◯**NO**
WHAT IS YOUR MOOD AFTER TREATMENT?

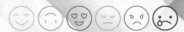

HOW DO YOU FEEL AFTER YOUR KETAMINE TREATMENT? DESCRIBE ANY CHANGES IN YOUR MOOD OR THOUGHTS.

WHAT INSIGHTS OR REALIZATIONS DID YOU HAVE DURING THE SESSION?

DATE: _____

KETAMINE DOSE: _____

WHAT IS YOUR MOOD GOING INTO THE TREATMENT?

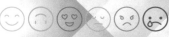

WHAT DID YOU EXPERIENCE DURING TREATMENT?

WHAT PHYSICAL SENSATIONS DID YOU NOTICE DURING YOUR TREATMENT? HOW DID THEY AFFECT YOU?

WHAT EMOTIONS SURFACED DURING THE SESSION? WERE THEY FAMILIAR OR NEW?

DID YOU EXPERIENCE ANY VISUAL CHANGES OR IMAGERY? DESCRIBE THEM IN DETAIL:

WHAT THOUGHTS OR MEMORIES CAME UP DURING YOUR TREATMENT? HOW DID YOU FEEL ABOUT THEM?

Post-Session Reflection

DID YOU DISASSOCIATE?   ◯YES   ◯NO
WHAT IS YOUR MOOD AFTER TREATMENT?

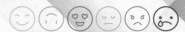

HOW DO YOU FEEL AFTER YOUR KETAMINE TREATMENT? DESCRIBE ANY CHANGES IN YOUR MOOD OR THOUGHTS.

WHAT INSIGHTS OR REALIZATIONS DID YOU HAVE DURING THE SESSION?

DATE: _____

KETAMINE DOSE: _____

WHAT IS YOUR MOOD GOING INTO THE TREATMENT?

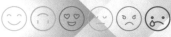

WHAT DID YOU EXPERIENCE DURING TREATMENT?

WHAT PHYSICAL SENSATIONS DID YOU NOTICE DURING YOUR
TREATMENT? HOW DID THEY AFFECT YOU?

WHAT EMOTIONS SURFACED DURING THE SESSION? WERE
THEY FAMILIAR OR NEW?

DID YOU EXPERIENCE ANY VISUAL CHANGES OR IMAGERY? DESCRIBE THEM IN DETAIL:

WHAT THOUGHTS OR MEMORIES CAME UP DURING YOUR TREATMENT? HOW DID YOU FEEL ABOUT THEM?

Post-Session Reflection

DID YOU DISASSOCIATE?   ○ YES   ○ NO

WHAT IS YOUR MOOD AFTER TREATMENT?

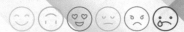

HOW DO YOU FEEL AFTER YOUR KETAMINE TREATMENT? DESCRIBE ANY CHANGES IN YOUR MOOD OR THOUGHTS.

WHAT INSIGHTS OR REALIZATIONS DID YOU HAVE DURING THE SESSION?

DATE: _____

KETAMINE DOSE: _____

WHAT IS YOUR MOOD GOING INTO THE TREATMENT?

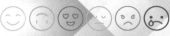

WHAT DID YOU EXPERIENCE DURING TREATMENT?

WHAT PHYSICAL SENSATIONS DID YOU NOTICE DURING YOUR TREATMENT? HOW DID THEY AFFECT YOU?

WHAT EMOTIONS SURFACED DURING THE SESSION? WERE THEY FAMILIAR OR NEW?

DID YOU EXPERIENCE ANY VISUAL CHANGES OR IMAGERY? DESCRIBE THEM IN DETAIL:

WHAT THOUGHTS OR MEMORIES CAME UP DURING YOUR TREATMENT? HOW DID YOU FEEL ABOUT THEM?

Post-Session Reflection

DID YOU DISASSOCIATE?   ◯YES   ◯NO
WHAT IS YOUR MOOD AFTER TREATMENT?

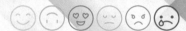

HOW DO YOU FEEL AFTER YOUR KETAMINE TREATMENT? DESCRIBE ANY CHANGES IN YOUR MOOD OR THOUGHTS.

WHAT INSIGHTS OR REALIZATIONS DID YOU HAVE DURING THE SESSION?

DATE: _____

KETAMINE DOSE: _____

WHAT IS YOUR MOOD GOING INTO THE TREATMENT?

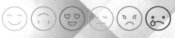

WHAT DID YOU EXPERIENCE DURING TREATMENT?

WHAT PHYSICAL SENSATIONS DID YOU NOTICE DURING YOUR
TREATMENT? HOW DID THEY AFFECT YOU?

WHAT EMOTIONS SURFACED DURING THE SESSION? WERE
THEY FAMILIAR OR NEW?

DID YOU EXPERIENCE ANY VISUAL CHANGES OR IMAGERY? DESCRIBE THEM IN DETAIL:

WHAT THOUGHTS OR MEMORIES CAME UP DURING YOUR TREATMENT? HOW DID YOU FEEL ABOUT THEM?

Post-Session Reflection

DID YOU DISASSOCIATE? ◯ YES ◯ NO

WHAT IS YOUR MOOD AFTER TREATMENT?

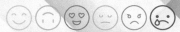

HOW DO YOU FEEL AFTER YOUR KETAMINE TREATMENT? DESCRIBE ANY CHANGES IN YOUR MOOD OR THOUGHTS.

WHAT INSIGHTS OR REALIZATIONS DID YOU HAVE DURING THE SESSION?

DATE: _____

KETAMINE DOSE: _____

WHAT IS YOUR MOOD GOING INTO THE TREATMENT?

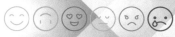

WHAT DID YOU EXPERIENCE DURING TREATMENT?

WHAT PHYSICAL SENSATIONS DID YOU NOTICE DURING YOUR TREATMENT? HOW DID THEY AFFECT YOU?

WHAT EMOTIONS SURFACED DURING THE SESSION? WERE THEY FAMILIAR OR NEW?

DID YOU EXPERIENCE ANY VISUAL CHANGES OR IMAGERY? DESCRIBE THEM IN DETAIL:

WHAT THOUGHTS OR MEMORIES CAME UP DURING YOUR TREATMENT? HOW DID YOU FEEL ABOUT THEM?

Post-Session Reflection

DID YOU DISASSOCIATE?   ◯ YES   ◯ NO

WHAT IS YOUR MOOD AFTER TREATMENT?

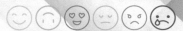

HOW DO YOU FEEL AFTER YOUR KETAMINE TREATMENT? DESCRIBE ANY CHANGES IN YOUR MOOD OR THOUGHTS.

WHAT INSIGHTS OR REALIZATIONS DID YOU HAVE DURING THE SESSION?

DATE: _____

KETAMINE DOSE: _____

WHAT IS YOUR MOOD GOING INTO THE TREATMENT?

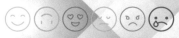

WHAT DID YOU EXPERIENCE DURING TREATMENT?

WHAT PHYSICAL SENSATIONS DID YOU NOTICE DURING YOUR
TREATMENT? HOW DID THEY AFFECT YOU?

WHAT EMOTIONS SURFACED DURING THE SESSION? WERE
THEY FAMILIAR OR NEW?

DID YOU EXPERIENCE ANY VISUAL CHANGES OR IMAGERY? DESCRIBE THEM IN DETAIL:

WHAT THOUGHTS OR MEMORIES CAME UP DURING YOUR TREATMENT? HOW DID YOU FEEL ABOUT THEM?

Post-Session Reflection

DID YOU DISASSOCIATE? ◯YES ◯NO
WHAT IS YOUR MOOD AFTER TREATMENT?

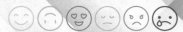

HOW DO YOU FEEL AFTER YOUR KETAMINE TREATMENT? DESCRIBE ANY CHANGES IN YOUR MOOD OR THOUGHTS.

WHAT INSIGHTS OR REALIZATIONS DID YOU HAVE DURING THE SESSION?

DATE: _____

KETAMINE DOSE: _____

WHAT IS YOUR MOOD GOING INTO THE TREATMENT?

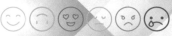

WHAT DID YOU EXPERIENCE DURING TREATMENT?

WHAT PHYSICAL SENSATIONS DID YOU NOTICE DURING YOUR TREATMENT? HOW DID THEY AFFECT YOU?

WHAT EMOTIONS SURFACED DURING THE SESSION? WERE THEY FAMILIAR OR NEW?

DID YOU EXPERIENCE ANY VISUAL CHANGES OR IMAGERY? DESCRIBE THEM IN DETAIL:

WHAT THOUGHTS OR MEMORIES CAME UP DURING YOUR TREATMENT? HOW DID YOU FEEL ABOUT THEM?

Post-Session Reflection

DID YOU DISASSOCIATE?   ◯ YES   ◯ NO
WHAT IS YOUR MOOD AFTER TREATMENT?

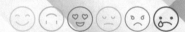

HOW DO YOU FEEL AFTER YOUR KETAMINE TREATMENT? DESCRIBE ANY CHANGES IN YOUR MOOD OR THOUGHTS.

WHAT INSIGHTS OR REALIZATIONS DID YOU HAVE DURING THE SESSION?

DATE: _____

KETAMINE DOSE: _____

WHAT IS YOUR MOOD GOING INTO THE TREATMENT?

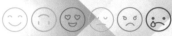

WHAT DID YOU EXPERIENCE DURING TREATMENT?

WHAT PHYSICAL SENSATIONS DID YOU NOTICE DURING YOUR
TREATMENT? HOW DID THEY AFFECT YOU?

WHAT EMOTIONS SURFACED DURING THE SESSION? WERE
THEY FAMILIAR OR NEW?

DID YOU EXPERIENCE ANY VISUAL CHANGES OR IMAGERY? DESCRIBE THEM IN DETAIL:

WHAT THOUGHTS OR MEMORIES CAME UP DURING YOUR TREATMENT? HOW DID YOU FEEL ABOUT THEM?

Post-Session Reflection

DID YOU DISASSOCIATE? ⚪YES ⚪NO
WHAT IS YOUR MOOD AFTER TREATMENT?

HOW DO YOU FEEL AFTER YOUR KETAMINE TREATMENT? DESCRIBE ANY CHANGES IN YOUR MOOD OR THOUGHTS.

WHAT INSIGHTS OR REALIZATIONS DID YOU HAVE DURING THE SESSION?

DATE: _____

KETAMINE DOSE: _____

WHAT IS YOUR MOOD GOING INTO THE TREATMENT?

WHAT DID YOU EXPERIENCE DURING TREATMENT?

WHAT PHYSICAL SENSATIONS DID YOU NOTICE DURING YOUR TREATMENT? HOW DID THEY AFFECT YOU?

WHAT EMOTIONS SURFACED DURING THE SESSION? WERE THEY FAMILIAR OR NEW?

**DID YOU EXPERIENCE ANY VISUAL CHANGES OR IMAGERY?
DESCRIBE THEM IN DETAIL:**

**WHAT THOUGHTS OR MEMORIES CAME UP DURING YOUR
TREATMENT? HOW DID YOU FEEL ABOUT THEM?**

Post-Session Reflection

**DID YOU DISASSOCIATE?   ◯ YES   ◯ NO
WHAT IS YOUR MOOD AFTER TREATMENT?**

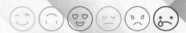

**HOW DO YOU FEEL AFTER YOUR KETAMINE TREATMENT?
DESCRIBE ANY CHANGES IN YOUR MOOD OR THOUGHTS.**

**WHAT INSIGHTS OR REALIZATIONS DID YOU HAVE DURING
THE SESSION?**

DATE: _____

KETAMINE DOSE: _____

WHAT IS YOUR MOOD GOING INTO THE TREATMENT?

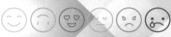

WHAT DID YOU EXPERIENCE DURING TREATMENT?

WHAT PHYSICAL SENSATIONS DID YOU NOTICE DURING YOUR TREATMENT? HOW DID THEY AFFECT YOU?

WHAT EMOTIONS SURFACED DURING THE SESSION? WERE THEY FAMILIAR OR NEW?

DID YOU EXPERIENCE ANY VISUAL CHANGES OR IMAGERY?
DESCRIBE THEM IN DETAIL:

WHAT THOUGHTS OR MEMORIES CAME UP DURING YOUR
TREATMENT? HOW DID YOU FEEL ABOUT THEM?

Post-Session Reflection

DID YOU DISASSOCIATE? ◯**YES**   ◯**NO**
WHAT IS YOUR MOOD AFTER TREATMENT?

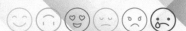

HOW DO YOU FEEL AFTER YOUR KETAMINE TREATMENT?
DESCRIBE ANY CHANGES IN YOUR MOOD OR THOUGHTS.

WHAT INSIGHTS OR REALIZATIONS DID YOU HAVE DURING
THE SESSION?

DATE: _____

KETAMINE DOSE: _____

WHAT IS YOUR MOOD GOING INTO THE TREATMENT?

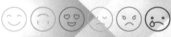

WHAT DID YOU EXPERIENCE DURING TREATMENT?

WHAT PHYSICAL SENSATIONS DID YOU NOTICE DURING YOUR TREATMENT? HOW DID THEY AFFECT YOU?

WHAT EMOTIONS SURFACED DURING THE SESSION? WERE THEY FAMILIAR OR NEW?

DID YOU EXPERIENCE ANY VISUAL CHANGES OR IMAGERY? DESCRIBE THEM IN DETAIL:

WHAT THOUGHTS OR MEMORIES CAME UP DURING YOUR TREATMENT? HOW DID YOU FEEL ABOUT THEM?

Post-Session Reflection

DID YOU DISASSOCIATE?   ◯YES   ◯NO
WHAT IS YOUR MOOD AFTER TREATMENT?

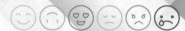

HOW DO YOU FEEL AFTER YOUR KETAMINE TREATMENT? DESCRIBE ANY CHANGES IN YOUR MOOD OR THOUGHTS.

WHAT INSIGHTS OR REALIZATIONS DID YOU HAVE DURING THE SESSION?

DATE: _____

KETAMINE DOSE: _____

WHAT IS YOUR MOOD GOING INTO THE TREATMENT?

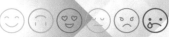

WHAT DID YOU EXPERIENCE DURING TREATMENT?

WHAT PHYSICAL SENSATIONS DID YOU NOTICE DURING YOUR
TREATMENT? HOW DID THEY AFFECT YOU?

WHAT EMOTIONS SURFACED DURING THE SESSION? WERE
THEY FAMILIAR OR NEW?

DID YOU EXPERIENCE ANY VISUAL CHANGES OR IMAGERY? DESCRIBE THEM IN DETAIL:

WHAT THOUGHTS OR MEMORIES CAME UP DURING YOUR TREATMENT? HOW DID YOU FEEL ABOUT THEM?

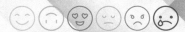

DID YOU DISASSOCIATE?   ◯YES   ◯NO
WHAT IS YOUR MOOD AFTER TREATMENT?

😊 🙂 😍 😞 😠 😢

HOW DO YOU FEEL AFTER YOUR KETAMINE TREATMENT? DESCRIBE ANY CHANGES IN YOUR MOOD OR THOUGHTS.

WHAT INSIGHTS OR REALIZATIONS DID YOU HAVE DURING THE SESSION?

DATE: _____

KETAMINE DOSE: _____

WHAT IS YOUR MOOD GOING INTO THE TREATMENT?

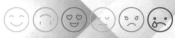

WHAT DID YOU EXPERIENCE DURING TREATMENT?

WHAT PHYSICAL SENSATIONS DID YOU NOTICE DURING YOUR TREATMENT? HOW DID THEY AFFECT YOU?

WHAT EMOTIONS SURFACED DURING THE SESSION? WERE THEY FAMILIAR OR NEW?

DID YOU EXPERIENCE ANY VISUAL CHANGES OR IMAGERY? DESCRIBE THEM IN DETAIL:

WHAT THOUGHTS OR MEMORIES CAME UP DURING YOUR TREATMENT? HOW DID YOU FEEL ABOUT THEM?

Post-Session Reflection

DID YOU DISASSOCIATE? ◯YES ◯NO
WHAT IS YOUR MOOD AFTER TREATMENT?

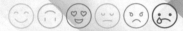

HOW DO YOU FEEL AFTER YOUR KETAMINE TREATMENT? DESCRIBE ANY CHANGES IN YOUR MOOD OR THOUGHTS.

WHAT INSIGHTS OR REALIZATIONS DID YOU HAVE DURING THE SESSION?

DATE: _____

KETAMINE DOSE: _____

WHAT IS YOUR MOOD GOING INTO THE TREATMENT?

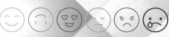

WHAT DID YOU EXPERIENCE DURING TREATMENT?

WHAT PHYSICAL SENSATIONS DID YOU NOTICE DURING YOUR TREATMENT? HOW DID THEY AFFECT YOU?

WHAT EMOTIONS SURFACED DURING THE SESSION? WERE THEY FAMILIAR OR NEW?

**DID YOU EXPERIENCE ANY VISUAL CHANGES OR IMAGERY?
DESCRIBE THEM IN DETAIL:**

**WHAT THOUGHTS OR MEMORIES CAME UP DURING YOUR
TREATMENT? HOW DID YOU FEEL ABOUT THEM?**

Post-Session Reflection

DID YOU DISASSOCIATE? ◯YES ◯NO
WHAT IS YOUR MOOD AFTER TREATMENT?

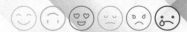

**HOW DO YOU FEEL AFTER YOUR KETAMINE TREATMENT?
DESCRIBE ANY CHANGES IN YOUR MOOD OR THOUGHTS.**

**WHAT INSIGHTS OR REALIZATIONS DID YOU HAVE DURING
THE SESSION?**

DATE: _____

KETAMINE DOSE: _____

WHAT IS YOUR MOOD GOING INTO THE TREATMENT?

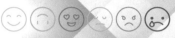

WHAT DID YOU EXPERIENCE DURING TREATMENT?

WHAT PHYSICAL SENSATIONS DID YOU NOTICE DURING YOUR
TREATMENT? HOW DID THEY AFFECT YOU?

WHAT EMOTIONS SURFACED DURING THE SESSION? WERE
THEY FAMILIAR OR NEW?

DID YOU EXPERIENCE ANY VISUAL CHANGES OR IMAGERY? DESCRIBE THEM IN DETAIL:

WHAT THOUGHTS OR MEMORIES CAME UP DURING YOUR TREATMENT? HOW DID YOU FEEL ABOUT THEM?

Post-Session Reflection

DID YOU DISASSOCIATE? ◯ YES ◯ NO
WHAT IS YOUR MOOD AFTER TREATMENT?

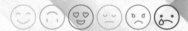

HOW DO YOU FEEL AFTER YOUR KETAMINE TREATMENT? DESCRIBE ANY CHANGES IN YOUR MOOD OR THOUGHTS.

WHAT INSIGHTS OR REALIZATIONS DID YOU HAVE DURING THE SESSION?

DATE: _____

KETAMINE DOSE: _____

WHAT IS YOUR MOOD GOING INTO THE TREATMENT?

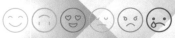

WHAT DID YOU EXPERIENCE DURING TREATMENT?

WHAT PHYSICAL SENSATIONS DID YOU NOTICE DURING YOUR TREATMENT? HOW DID THEY AFFECT YOU?

WHAT EMOTIONS SURFACED DURING THE SESSION? WERE THEY FAMILIAR OR NEW?

DID YOU EXPERIENCE ANY VISUAL CHANGES OR IMAGERY? DESCRIBE THEM IN DETAIL:

WHAT THOUGHTS OR MEMORIES CAME UP DURING YOUR TREATMENT? HOW DID YOU FEEL ABOUT THEM?

Post-Session Reflection

DID YOU DISASSOCIATE? ◯**YES** ◯**NO**

WHAT IS YOUR MOOD AFTER TREATMENT?

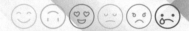

HOW DO YOU FEEL AFTER YOUR KETAMINE TREATMENT? DESCRIBE ANY CHANGES IN YOUR MOOD OR THOUGHTS.

WHAT INSIGHTS OR REALIZATIONS DID YOU HAVE DURING THE SESSION?

DATE: _____

KETAMINE DOSE: _____

WHAT IS YOUR MOOD GOING INTO THE TREATMENT?

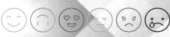

WHAT DID YOU EXPERIENCE DURING TREATMENT?

WHAT PHYSICAL SENSATIONS DID YOU NOTICE DURING YOUR TREATMENT? HOW DID THEY AFFECT YOU?

WHAT EMOTIONS SURFACED DURING THE SESSION? WERE THEY FAMILIAR OR NEW?

DID YOU EXPERIENCE ANY VISUAL CHANGES OR IMAGERY? DESCRIBE THEM IN DETAIL:

WHAT THOUGHTS OR MEMORIES CAME UP DURING YOUR TREATMENT? HOW DID YOU FEEL ABOUT THEM?

Post-Session Reflection

DID YOU DISASSOCIATE?   ◯YES   ◯NO
WHAT IS YOUR MOOD AFTER TREATMENT?

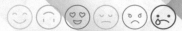

HOW DO YOU FEEL AFTER YOUR KETAMINE TREATMENT? DESCRIBE ANY CHANGES IN YOUR MOOD OR THOUGHTS.

WHAT INSIGHTS OR REALIZATIONS DID YOU HAVE DURING THE SESSION?

DATE: _____

KETAMINE DOSE: _____

WHAT IS YOUR MOOD GOING INTO THE TREATMENT?

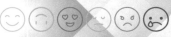

WHAT DID YOU EXPERIENCE DURING TREATMENT?

WHAT PHYSICAL SENSATIONS DID YOU NOTICE DURING YOUR TREATMENT? HOW DID THEY AFFECT YOU?

WHAT EMOTIONS SURFACED DURING THE SESSION? WERE THEY FAMILIAR OR NEW?

DID YOU EXPERIENCE ANY VISUAL CHANGES OR IMAGERY? DESCRIBE THEM IN DETAIL:

WHAT THOUGHTS OR MEMORIES CAME UP DURING YOUR TREATMENT? HOW DID YOU FEEL ABOUT THEM?

Post-Session Reflection

DID YOU DISASSOCIATE? ◯ **YES** ◯ **NO**

WHAT IS YOUR MOOD AFTER TREATMENT?

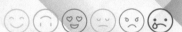

HOW DO YOU FEEL AFTER YOUR KETAMINE TREATMENT? DESCRIBE ANY CHANGES IN YOUR MOOD OR THOUGHTS.

WHAT INSIGHTS OR REALIZATIONS DID YOU HAVE DURING THE SESSION?

DATE: _____

KETAMINE DOSE: _____

WHAT IS YOUR MOOD GOING INTO THE TREATMENT?

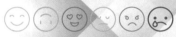

WHAT DID YOU EXPERIENCE DURING TREATMENT?

WHAT PHYSICAL SENSATIONS DID YOU NOTICE DURING YOUR TREATMENT? HOW DID THEY AFFECT YOU?

WHAT EMOTIONS SURFACED DURING THE SESSION? WERE THEY FAMILIAR OR NEW?

DID YOU EXPERIENCE ANY VISUAL CHANGES OR IMAGERY? DESCRIBE THEM IN DETAIL:

WHAT THOUGHTS OR MEMORIES CAME UP DURING YOUR TREATMENT? HOW DID YOU FEEL ABOUT THEM?

Post-Session Reflection

DID YOU DISASSOCIATE?   ◯**YES**   ◯**NO**

WHAT IS YOUR MOOD AFTER TREATMENT?

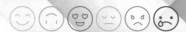

HOW DO YOU FEEL AFTER YOUR KETAMINE TREATMENT? DESCRIBE ANY CHANGES IN YOUR MOOD OR THOUGHTS.

WHAT INSIGHTS OR REALIZATIONS DID YOU HAVE DURING THE SESSION?

DATE: _____

KETAMINE DOSE: _____

WHAT IS YOUR MOOD GOING INTO THE TREATMENT?

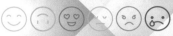

WHAT DID YOU EXPERIENCE DURING TREATMENT?

WHAT PHYSICAL SENSATIONS DID YOU NOTICE DURING YOUR
TREATMENT? HOW DID THEY AFFECT YOU?

WHAT EMOTIONS SURFACED DURING THE SESSION? WERE
THEY FAMILIAR OR NEW?

DID YOU EXPERIENCE ANY VISUAL CHANGES OR IMAGERY? DESCRIBE THEM IN DETAIL:

WHAT THOUGHTS OR MEMORIES CAME UP DURING YOUR TREATMENT? HOW DID YOU FEEL ABOUT THEM?

Post-Session Reflection

DID YOU DISASSOCIATE?   ◯ YES   ◯ NO

WHAT IS YOUR MOOD AFTER TREATMENT?

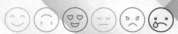

HOW DO YOU FEEL AFTER YOUR KETAMINE TREATMENT? DESCRIBE ANY CHANGES IN YOUR MOOD OR THOUGHTS.

WHAT INSIGHTS OR REALIZATIONS DID YOU HAVE DURING THE SESSION?

DATE: _____

KETAMINE DOSE: _____

WHAT IS YOUR MOOD GOING INTO THE TREATMENT?

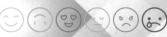

WHAT DID YOU EXPERIENCE DURING TREATMENT?

WHAT PHYSICAL SENSATIONS DID YOU NOTICE DURING YOUR TREATMENT? HOW DID THEY AFFECT YOU?

WHAT EMOTIONS SURFACED DURING THE SESSION? WERE THEY FAMILIAR OR NEW?

DID YOU EXPERIENCE ANY VISUAL CHANGES OR IMAGERY? DESCRIBE THEM IN DETAIL:

WHAT THOUGHTS OR MEMORIES CAME UP DURING YOUR TREATMENT? HOW DID YOU FEEL ABOUT THEM?

Post-Session Reflection

DID YOU DISASSOCIATE? ○ YES ○ NO
WHAT IS YOUR MOOD AFTER TREATMENT?

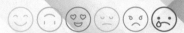

HOW DO YOU FEEL AFTER YOUR KETAMINE TREATMENT? DESCRIBE ANY CHANGES IN YOUR MOOD OR THOUGHTS.

WHAT INSIGHTS OR REALIZATIONS DID YOU HAVE DURING THE SESSION?

DATE: _____

KETAMINE DOSE: _____

WHAT IS YOUR MOOD GOING INTO THE TREATMENT?

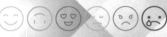

WHAT DID YOU EXPERIENCE DURING TREATMENT?

WHAT PHYSICAL SENSATIONS DID YOU NOTICE DURING YOUR TREATMENT? HOW DID THEY AFFECT YOU?

WHAT EMOTIONS SURFACED DURING THE SESSION? WERE THEY FAMILIAR OR NEW?

**DID YOU EXPERIENCE ANY VISUAL CHANGES OR IMAGERY?
DESCRIBE THEM IN DETAIL:**

**WHAT THOUGHTS OR MEMORIES CAME UP DURING YOUR
TREATMENT? HOW DID YOU FEEL ABOUT THEM?**

Post-Session Reflection

**DID YOU DISASSOCIATE?   ◯YES   ◯NO
WHAT IS YOUR MOOD AFTER TREATMENT?**

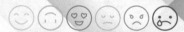

**HOW DO YOU FEEL AFTER YOUR KETAMINE TREATMENT?
DESCRIBE ANY CHANGES IN YOUR MOOD OR THOUGHTS.**

**WHAT INSIGHTS OR REALIZATIONS DID YOU HAVE DURING
THE SESSION?**

DATE: _____

KETAMINE DOSE: _____

WHAT IS YOUR MOOD GOING INTO THE TREATMENT?

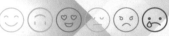

WHAT DID YOU EXPERIENCE DURING TREATMENT?

WHAT PHYSICAL SENSATIONS DID YOU NOTICE DURING YOUR TREATMENT? HOW DID THEY AFFECT YOU?

WHAT EMOTIONS SURFACED DURING THE SESSION? WERE THEY FAMILIAR OR NEW?

**DID YOU EXPERIENCE ANY VISUAL CHANGES OR IMAGERY?
DESCRIBE THEM IN DETAIL:**

**WHAT THOUGHTS OR MEMORIES CAME UP DURING YOUR
TREATMENT? HOW DID YOU FEEL ABOUT THEM?**

Post-Session Reflection

**DID YOU DISASSOCIATE?   ◯ YES   ◯ NO
WHAT IS YOUR MOOD AFTER TREATMENT?**

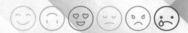

**HOW DO YOU FEEL AFTER YOUR KETAMINE TREATMENT?
DESCRIBE ANY CHANGES IN YOUR MOOD OR THOUGHTS.**

**WHAT INSIGHTS OR REALIZATIONS DID YOU HAVE DURING
THE SESSION?**

DATE: _____

KETAMINE DOSE: _____

WHAT IS YOUR MOOD GOING INTO THE TREATMENT?

WHAT DID YOU EXPERIENCE DURING TREATMENT?

WHAT PHYSICAL SENSATIONS DID YOU NOTICE DURING YOUR TREATMENT? HOW DID THEY AFFECT YOU?

WHAT EMOTIONS SURFACED DURING THE SESSION? WERE THEY FAMILIAR OR NEW?

**DID YOU EXPERIENCE ANY VISUAL CHANGES OR IMAGERY?
DESCRIBE THEM IN DETAIL:**

**WHAT THOUGHTS OR MEMORIES CAME UP DURING YOUR
TREATMENT? HOW DID YOU FEEL ABOUT THEM?**

Post-Session Reflection

**DID YOU DISASSOCIATE?   ○YES   ○NO
WHAT IS YOUR MOOD AFTER TREATMENT?**

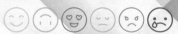

**HOW DO YOU FEEL AFTER YOUR KETAMINE TREATMENT?
DESCRIBE ANY CHANGES IN YOUR MOOD OR THOUGHTS.**

**WHAT INSIGHTS OR REALIZATIONS DID YOU HAVE DURING
THE SESSION?**

DATE: _____

KETAMINE DOSE: _____

WHAT IS YOUR MOOD GOING INTO THE TREATMENT?

WHAT DID YOU EXPERIENCE DURING TREATMENT?

WHAT PHYSICAL SENSATIONS DID YOU NOTICE DURING YOUR
TREATMENT? HOW DID THEY AFFECT YOU?

WHAT EMOTIONS SURFACED DURING THE SESSION? WERE
THEY FAMILIAR OR NEW?

DID YOU EXPERIENCE ANY VISUAL CHANGES OR IMAGERY? DESCRIBE THEM IN DETAIL:

WHAT THOUGHTS OR MEMORIES CAME UP DURING YOUR TREATMENT? HOW DID YOU FEEL ABOUT THEM?

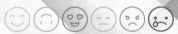

DID YOU DISASSOCIATE? ◯ YES   ◯ NO

WHAT IS YOUR MOOD AFTER TREATMENT?

😊 🙂 😍 😔 😠 🤕

HOW DO YOU FEEL AFTER YOUR KETAMINE TREATMENT? DESCRIBE ANY CHANGES IN YOUR MOOD OR THOUGHTS.

WHAT INSIGHTS OR REALIZATIONS DID YOU HAVE DURING THE SESSION?

DATE: _____

KETAMINE DOSE: _____

WHAT IS YOUR MOOD GOING INTO THE TREATMENT?

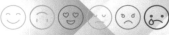

WHAT DID YOU EXPERIENCE DURING TREATMENT?

WHAT PHYSICAL SENSATIONS DID YOU NOTICE DURING YOUR TREATMENT? HOW DID THEY AFFECT YOU?

WHAT EMOTIONS SURFACED DURING THE SESSION? WERE THEY FAMILIAR OR NEW?

**DID YOU EXPERIENCE ANY VISUAL CHANGES OR IMAGERY?
DESCRIBE THEM IN DETAIL:**

**WHAT THOUGHTS OR MEMORIES CAME UP DURING YOUR
TREATMENT? HOW DID YOU FEEL ABOUT THEM?**

Post-Session Reflection

**DID YOU DISASSOCIATE?   ◯YES   ◯NO
WHAT IS YOUR MOOD AFTER TREATMENT?**

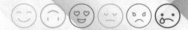

**HOW DO YOU FEEL AFTER YOUR KETAMINE TREATMENT?
DESCRIBE ANY CHANGES IN YOUR MOOD OR THOUGHTS.**

**WHAT INSIGHTS OR REALIZATIONS DID YOU HAVE DURING
THE SESSION?**

DATE: _____

KETAMINE DOSE: _____

WHAT IS YOUR MOOD GOING INTO THE TREATMENT?

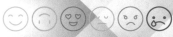

WHAT DID YOU EXPERIENCE DURING TREATMENT?

WHAT PHYSICAL SENSATIONS DID YOU NOTICE DURING YOUR TREATMENT? HOW DID THEY AFFECT YOU?

WHAT EMOTIONS SURFACED DURING THE SESSION? WERE THEY FAMILIAR OR NEW?

DID YOU EXPERIENCE ANY VISUAL CHANGES OR IMAGERY? DESCRIBE THEM IN DETAIL:

WHAT THOUGHTS OR MEMORIES CAME UP DURING YOUR TREATMENT? HOW DID YOU FEEL ABOUT THEM?

Post-Session Reflection

DID YOU DISASSOCIATE?   ◯ **YES**   ◯ **NO**
WHAT IS YOUR MOOD AFTER TREATMENT?

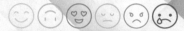

HOW DO YOU FEEL AFTER YOUR KETAMINE TREATMENT? DESCRIBE ANY CHANGES IN YOUR MOOD OR THOUGHTS.

WHAT INSIGHTS OR REALIZATIONS DID YOU HAVE DURING THE SESSION?

DATE: _____

KETAMINE DOSE: _____

WHAT IS YOUR MOOD GOING INTO THE TREATMENT?

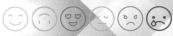

WHAT DID YOU EXPERIENCE DURING TREATMENT?

WHAT PHYSICAL SENSATIONS DID YOU NOTICE DURING YOUR
TREATMENT? HOW DID THEY AFFECT YOU?

WHAT EMOTIONS SURFACED DURING THE SESSION? WERE
THEY FAMILIAR OR NEW?

DID YOU EXPERIENCE ANY VISUAL CHANGES OR IMAGERY? DESCRIBE THEM IN DETAIL:

WHAT THOUGHTS OR MEMORIES CAME UP DURING YOUR TREATMENT? HOW DID YOU FEEL ABOUT THEM?

Post-Session Reflection

DID YOU DISASSOCIATE? ⭘YES ⭘NO

WHAT IS YOUR MOOD AFTER TREATMENT?

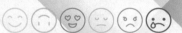

HOW DO YOU FEEL AFTER YOUR KETAMINE TREATMENT? DESCRIBE ANY CHANGES IN YOUR MOOD OR THOUGHTS.

WHAT INSIGHTS OR REALIZATIONS DID YOU HAVE DURING THE SESSION?

DATE: _____

KETAMINE DOSE: _____

WHAT IS YOUR MOOD GOING INTO THE TREATMENT?

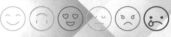

WHAT DID YOU EXPERIENCE DURING TREATMENT?

WHAT PHYSICAL SENSATIONS DID YOU NOTICE DURING YOUR
TREATMENT? HOW DID THEY AFFECT YOU?

WHAT EMOTIONS SURFACED DURING THE SESSION? WERE
THEY FAMILIAR OR NEW?

DID YOU EXPERIENCE ANY VISUAL CHANGES OR IMAGERY? DESCRIBE THEM IN DETAIL:

WHAT THOUGHTS OR MEMORIES CAME UP DURING YOUR TREATMENT? HOW DID YOU FEEL ABOUT THEM?

Post-Session Reflection

DID YOU DISASSOCIATE? ⃝ **YES** ⃝ **NO**
WHAT IS YOUR MOOD AFTER TREATMENT?

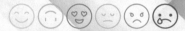

HOW DO YOU FEEL AFTER YOUR KETAMINE TREATMENT? DESCRIBE ANY CHANGES IN YOUR MOOD OR THOUGHTS.

WHAT INSIGHTS OR REALIZATIONS DID YOU HAVE DURING THE SESSION?

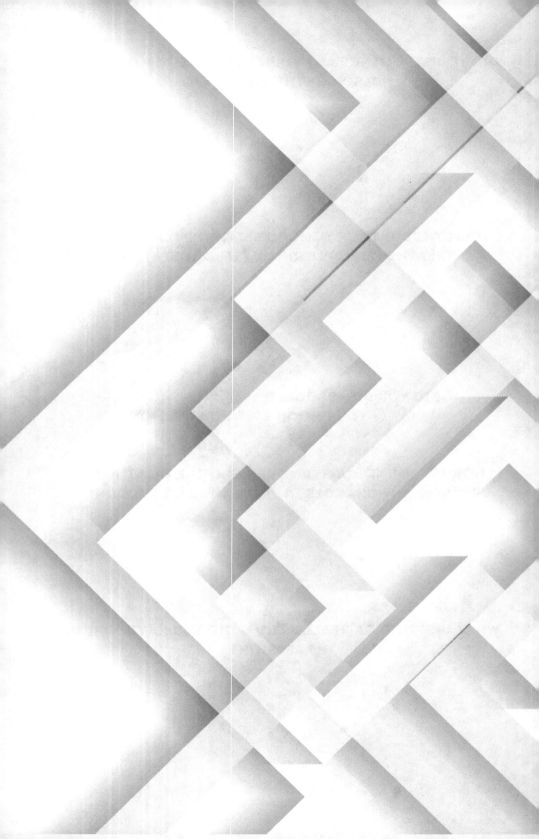

Between Treatment Reflection

Between Session Reflection

HOW ARE YOU INTEGRATING THE EXPERIENCES FROM YOUR KETAMINE SESSIONS INTO YOUR DAILY LIFE?

HAVE YOU NOTICED ANY CHANGES IN YOUR THOUGHTS OR EMOTIONS BETWEEN SESSIONS?

HAVE YOU NOTICED ANY CHANGES IN YOUR HABITS OR BEHAVIORS?

ARE THERE ACTIVITIES OR TASKS THAT YOUR FIND EASIER OR
MORE DIFFICULT NOW?

HAVE YOU FELT MORE MOTIVATED OR LESS MOTIVATED TO
ENGAGE IN CERTAIN ACTIVITIES?

WHAT SELF-CARE PRACTICES ARE YOU INCORPORATING TO
SUPPORT YOUR TREATMENT? HOW ARE THEY HELPING YOU?

WHO IN YOUR LIFE IS PROVIDING SUPPORT DURING THIS TREATMENT? HOW ARE THEY HELPING YOU?

HOW HAVE YOUR INTERACTIONS WITH OTHERS BEEN SINCE YOU STARTED TREATMENT?

HAVE YOU NOTICED ANY CHANGES IN YOUR COMMUNICATION OR RELATIONSHIPS WITH FAMILY, FRIENDS, OR COLLEAGUES?

WHAT ARE YOUR GOALS OR INTENTIONS FOR YOUR FUTURE KETAMINE SESSIONS?

HIS THERE ANYTHING SPECIFIC YOU WOULD LIKE TO FOCUS ON OR EXPLORE FURTHER?

HOW DO YOU HOPE TO CONTINUE GROWING OR HEALING THROUGH FUTURE SESSIONS?

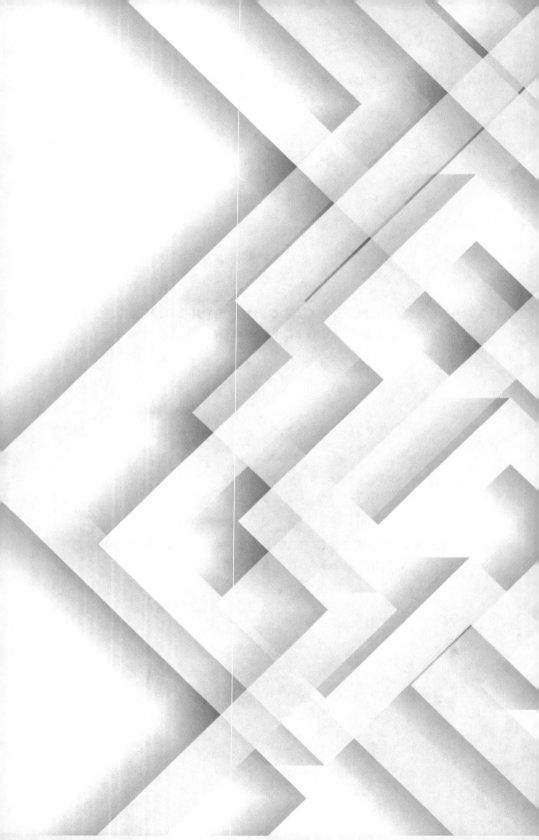

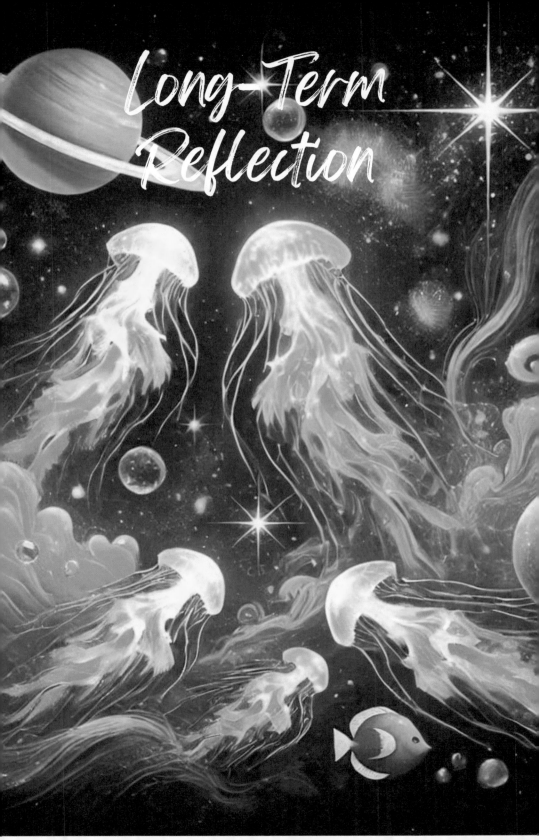

Long-Term
Reflection

Long-Term Reflections

REFLECT ON YOUR PROGRESS SINCE STARTING KETAMINE TREATMENT. WHAT CHANGES HAVE YOU NOTICED IN YOURSELF?

WHAT IMPROVEMENTS OR CHALLENGES HAVE YOU EXPERIENCED ALONG THE WAY?

WHAT ARE YOUR GOALS FOR THE FUTURE AFTER COMPLETING KETAMINE TREATMENT?

HOW DO YOU PLAN TO MAINTAIN THE POSITIVE CHANGES YOU'VE EXPERIENCED?

WRITE ABOUT THREE THINGS YOU ARE GRATEFUL FOR FROM TREATMENT. HOW DO THEY IMPACT YOUR OVERALL WELL-BEING?

DESCRIBE A POSITIVE EXPERIENCE OR MOMENT FROM YOUR TREATMENT. HOW DID IT MAKE YOU FEEL?"

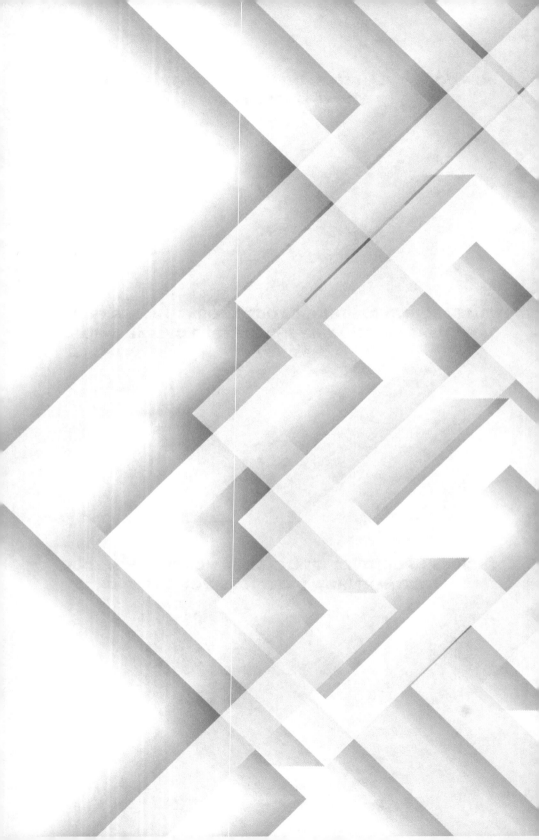

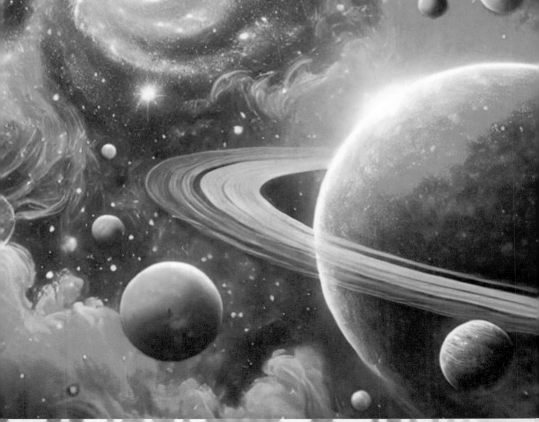

Emotional Check-In

DATE: _____

HOW ARE YOU FEELING TODAY? WHAT EMOTIONS ARE YOU EXPERIENCING?

WHAT STRATEGIES CAN YOU USE TO MANAGE ANY DIFFICULT EMOTIONS YOU ARE FACING?

SPEND A FEW MOMENTS IN MINDFULNESS. WHAT THOUGHTS AND FEELINGS COME UP DURING THIS TIME?

HOW CAN YOU INCORPORATE MINDFULNESS INTO YOUR DAILY ROUTINE TO SUPPORT YOUR TREATMENT?

DATE: _____

HOW ARE YOU FEELING TODAY? WHAT EMOTIONS ARE YOU EXPERIENCING?

WHAT STRATEGIES CAN YOU USE TO MANAGE ANY DIFFICULT EMOTIONS YOU ARE FACING?

SPEND A FEW MOMENTS IN MINDFULNESS. WHAT THOUGHTS AND FEELINGS COME UP DURING THIS TIME?

HOW CAN YOU INCORPORATE MINDFULNESS INTO YOUR DAILY ROUTINE TO SUPPORT YOUR TREATMENT?

DATE: _____

HOW ARE YOU FEELING TODAY? WHAT EMOTIONS ARE YOU EXPERIENCING?

WHAT STRATEGIES CAN YOU USE TO MANAGE ANY DIFFICULT EMOTIONS YOU ARE FACING?

SPEND A FEW MOMENTS IN MINDFULNESS. WHAT THOUGHTS AND FEELINGS COME UP DURING THIS TIME?

HOW CAN YOU INCORPORATE MINDFULNESS INTO YOUR DAILY ROUTINE TO SUPPORT YOUR TREATMENT?

DATE: _____

HOW ARE YOU FEELING TODAY? WHAT EMOTIONS ARE
YOU EXPERIENCING?

WHAT STRATEGIES CAN YOU USE TO MANAGE ANY
DIFFICULT EMOTIONS YOU ARE FACING?

SPEND A FEW MOMENTS IN MINDFULNESS. WHAT
THOUGHTS AND FEELINGS COME UP DURING THIS TIME?

HOW CAN YOU INCORPORATE MINDFULNESS INTO YOUR
DAILY ROUTINE TO SUPPORT YOUR TREATMENT?

DATE: _____

HOW ARE YOU FEELING TODAY? WHAT EMOTIONS ARE YOU EXPERIENCING?

WHAT STRATEGIES CAN YOU USE TO MANAGE ANY DIFFICULT EMOTIONS YOU ARE FACING?

SPEND A FEW MOMENTS IN MINDFULNESS. WHAT THOUGHTS AND FEELINGS COME UP DURING THIS TIME?

HOW CAN YOU INCORPORATE MINDFULNESS INTO YOUR DAILY ROUTINE TO SUPPORT YOUR TREATMENT?

DATE: _____

HOW ARE YOU FEELING TODAY? WHAT EMOTIONS ARE YOU EXPERIENCING?

WHAT STRATEGIES CAN YOU USE TO MANAGE ANY DIFFICULT EMOTIONS YOU ARE FACING?

SPEND A FEW MOMENTS IN MINDFULNESS. WHAT THOUGHTS AND FEELINGS COME UP DURING THIS TIME?

HOW CAN YOU INCORPORATE MINDFULNESS INTO YOUR DAILY ROUTINE TO SUPPORT YOUR TREATMENT?

DATE: _____

HOW ARE YOU FEELING TODAY? WHAT EMOTIONS ARE YOU EXPERIENCING?

WHAT STRATEGIES CAN YOU USE TO MANAGE ANY DIFFICULT EMOTIONS YOU ARE FACING?

SPEND A FEW MOMENTS IN MINDFULNESS. WHAT THOUGHTS AND FEELINGS COME UP DURING THIS TIME?

HOW CAN YOU INCORPORATE MINDFULNESS INTO YOUR DAILY ROUTINE TO SUPPORT YOUR TREATMENT?

DATE: _____

HOW ARE YOU FEELING TODAY? WHAT EMOTIONS ARE YOU EXPERIENCING?

WHAT STRATEGIES CAN YOU USE TO MANAGE ANY DIFFICULT EMOTIONS YOU ARE FACING?

SPEND A FEW MOMENTS IN MINDFULNESS. WHAT THOUGHTS AND FEELINGS COME UP DURING THIS TIME?

HOW CAN YOU INCORPORATE MINDFULNESS INTO YOUR DAILY ROUTINE TO SUPPORT YOUR TREATMENT?

DATE: _____

HOW ARE YOU FEELING TODAY? WHAT EMOTIONS ARE YOU EXPERIENCING?

WHAT STRATEGIES CAN YOU USE TO MANAGE ANY DIFFICULT EMOTIONS YOU ARE FACING?

SPEND A FEW MOMENTS IN MINDFULNESS. WHAT THOUGHTS AND FEELINGS COME UP DURING THIS TIME?

HOW CAN YOU INCORPORATE MINDFULNESS INTO YOUR DAILY ROUTINE TO SUPPORT YOUR TREATMENT?

DATE: _____

HOW ARE YOU FEELING TODAY? WHAT EMOTIONS ARE YOU EXPERIENCING?

WHAT STRATEGIES CAN YOU USE TO MANAGE ANY DIFFICULT EMOTIONS YOU ARE FACING?

SPEND A FEW MOMENTS IN MINDFULNESS. WHAT THOUGHTS AND FEELINGS COME UP DURING THIS TIME?

HOW CAN YOU INCORPORATE MINDFULNESS INTO YOUR DAILY ROUTINE TO SUPPORT YOUR TREATMENT?

DATE: _____

HOW ARE YOU FEELING TODAY? WHAT EMOTIONS ARE YOU EXPERIENCING?

WHAT STRATEGIES CAN YOU USE TO MANAGE ANY DIFFICULT EMOTIONS YOU ARE FACING?

SPEND A FEW MOMENTS IN MINDFULNESS. WHAT THOUGHTS AND FEELINGS COME UP DURING THIS TIME?

HOW CAN YOU INCORPORATE MINDFULNESS INTO YOUR DAILY ROUTINE TO SUPPORT YOUR TREATMENT?

DATE: _____

HOW ARE YOU FEELING TODAY? WHAT EMOTIONS ARE YOU EXPERIENCING?

WHAT STRATEGIES CAN YOU USE TO MANAGE ANY DIFFICULT EMOTIONS YOU ARE FACING?

SPEND A FEW MOMENTS IN MINDFULNESS. WHAT THOUGHTS AND FEELINGS COME UP DURING THIS TIME?

HOW CAN YOU INCORPORATE MINDFULNESS INTO YOUR DAILY ROUTINE TO SUPPORT YOUR TREATMENT?

DATE: _____

HOW ARE YOU FEELING TODAY? WHAT EMOTIONS ARE YOU EXPERIENCING?

WHAT STRATEGIES CAN YOU USE TO MANAGE ANY DIFFICULT EMOTIONS YOU ARE FACING?

SPEND A FEW MOMENTS IN MINDFULNESS. WHAT THOUGHTS AND FEELINGS COME UP DURING THIS TIME?

HOW CAN YOU INCORPORATE MINDFULNESS INTO YOUR DAILY ROUTINE TO SUPPORT YOUR TREATMENT?

DATE: _____

HOW ARE YOU FEELING TODAY? WHAT EMOTIONS ARE YOU EXPERIENCING?

WHAT STRATEGIES CAN YOU USE TO MANAGE ANY DIFFICULT EMOTIONS YOU ARE FACING?

SPEND A FEW MOMENTS IN MINDFULNESS. WHAT THOUGHTS AND FEELINGS COME UP DURING THIS TIME?

HOW CAN YOU INCORPORATE MINDFULNESS INTO YOUR DAILY ROUTINE TO SUPPORT YOUR TREATMENT?

DATE: _____

HOW ARE YOU FEELING TODAY? WHAT EMOTIONS ARE YOU EXPERIENCING?

WHAT STRATEGIES CAN YOU USE TO MANAGE ANY DIFFICULT EMOTIONS YOU ARE FACING?

SPEND A FEW MOMENTS IN MINDFULNESS. WHAT THOUGHTS AND FEELINGS COME UP DURING THIS TIME?

HOW CAN YOU INCORPORATE MINDFULNESS INTO YOUR DAILY ROUTINE TO SUPPORT YOUR TREATMENT?

DATE: _____

HOW ARE YOU FEELING TODAY? WHAT EMOTIONS ARE YOU EXPERIENCING?

WHAT STRATEGIES CAN YOU USE TO MANAGE ANY DIFFICULT EMOTIONS YOU ARE FACING?

SPEND A FEW MOMENTS IN MINDFULNESS. WHAT THOUGHTS AND FEELINGS COME UP DURING THIS TIME?

HOW CAN YOU INCORPORATE MINDFULNESS INTO YOUR DAILY ROUTINE TO SUPPORT YOUR TREATMENT?

DATE: _____

HOW ARE YOU FEELING TODAY? WHAT EMOTIONS ARE YOU EXPERIENCING?

WHAT STRATEGIES CAN YOU USE TO MANAGE ANY DIFFICULT EMOTIONS YOU ARE FACING?

SPEND A FEW MOMENTS IN MINDFULNESS. WHAT THOUGHTS AND FEELINGS COME UP DURING THIS TIME?

HOW CAN YOU INCORPORATE MINDFULNESS INTO YOUR DAILY ROUTINE TO SUPPORT YOUR TREATMENT?

DATE: _____

HOW ARE YOU FEELING TODAY? WHAT EMOTIONS ARE YOU EXPERIENCING?

WHAT STRATEGIES CAN YOU USE TO MANAGE ANY DIFFICULT EMOTIONS YOU ARE FACING?

SPEND A FEW MOMENTS IN MINDFULNESS. WHAT THOUGHTS AND FEELINGS COME UP DURING THIS TIME?

HOW CAN YOU INCORPORATE MINDFULNESS INTO YOUR DAILY ROUTINE TO SUPPORT YOUR TREATMENT?

DATE: _____

HOW ARE YOU FEELING TODAY? WHAT EMOTIONS ARE YOU EXPERIENCING?

WHAT STRATEGIES CAN YOU USE TO MANAGE ANY DIFFICULT EMOTIONS YOU ARE FACING?

SPEND A FEW MOMENTS IN MINDFULNESS. WHAT THOUGHTS AND FEELINGS COME UP DURING THIS TIME?

HOW CAN YOU INCORPORATE MINDFULNESS INTO YOUR DAILY ROUTINE TO SUPPORT YOUR TREATMENT?

DATE: _____

HOW ARE YOU FEELING TODAY? WHAT EMOTIONS ARE YOU EXPERIENCING?

WHAT STRATEGIES CAN YOU USE TO MANAGE ANY DIFFICULT EMOTIONS YOU ARE FACING?

SPEND A FEW MOMENTS IN MINDFULNESS. WHAT THOUGHTS AND FEELINGS COME UP DURING THIS TIME?

HOW CAN YOU INCORPORATE MINDFULNESS INTO YOUR DAILY ROUTINE TO SUPPORT YOUR TREATMENT?

DATE: _____

HOW ARE YOU FEELING TODAY? WHAT EMOTIONS ARE YOU EXPERIENCING?

WHAT STRATEGIES CAN YOU USE TO MANAGE ANY DIFFICULT EMOTIONS YOU ARE FACING?

SPEND A FEW MOMENTS IN MINDFULNESS. WHAT THOUGHTS AND FEELINGS COME UP DURING THIS TIME?

HOW CAN YOU INCORPORATE MINDFULNESS INTO YOUR DAILY ROUTINE TO SUPPORT YOUR TREATMENT?

DATE: _____

HOW ARE YOU FEELING TODAY? WHAT EMOTIONS ARE YOU EXPERIENCING?

WHAT STRATEGIES CAN YOU USE TO MANAGE ANY DIFFICULT EMOTIONS YOU ARE FACING?

SPEND A FEW MOMENTS IN MINDFULNESS. WHAT THOUGHTS AND FEELINGS COME UP DURING THIS TIME?

HOW CAN YOU INCORPORATE MINDFULNESS INTO YOUR DAILY ROUTINE TO SUPPORT YOUR TREATMENT?

DATE: _____

HOW ARE YOU FEELING TODAY? WHAT EMOTIONS ARE YOU EXPERIENCING?

WHAT STRATEGIES CAN YOU USE TO MANAGE ANY DIFFICULT EMOTIONS YOU ARE FACING?

SPEND A FEW MOMENTS IN MINDFULNESS. WHAT THOUGHTS AND FEELINGS COME UP DURING THIS TIME?

HOW CAN YOU INCORPORATE MINDFULNESS INTO YOUR DAILY ROUTINE TO SUPPORT YOUR TREATMENT?

DATE: _____

HOW ARE YOU FEELING TODAY? WHAT EMOTIONS ARE YOU EXPERIENCING?

WHAT STRATEGIES CAN YOU USE TO MANAGE ANY DIFFICULT EMOTIONS YOU ARE FACING?

SPEND A FEW MOMENTS IN MINDFULNESS. WHAT THOUGHTS AND FEELINGS COME UP DURING THIS TIME?

HOW CAN YOU INCORPORATE MINDFULNESS INTO YOUR DAILY ROUTINE TO SUPPORT YOUR TREATMENT?

DATE: _____

HOW ARE YOU FEELING TODAY? WHAT EMOTIONS ARE YOU EXPERIENCING?

WHAT STRATEGIES CAN YOU USE TO MANAGE ANY DIFFICULT EMOTIONS YOU ARE FACING?

SPEND A FEW MOMENTS IN MINDFULNESS. WHAT THOUGHTS AND FEELINGS COME UP DURING THIS TIME?

HOW CAN YOU INCORPORATE MINDFULNESS INTO YOUR DAILY ROUTINE TO SUPPORT YOUR TREATMENT?

DATE: _____

HOW ARE YOU FEELING TODAY? WHAT EMOTIONS ARE
YOU EXPERIENCING?

WHAT STRATEGIES CAN YOU USE TO MANAGE ANY
DIFFICULT EMOTIONS YOU ARE FACING?

SPEND A FEW MOMENTS IN MINDFULNESS. WHAT
THOUGHTS AND FEELINGS COME UP DURING THIS TIME?

HOW CAN YOU INCORPORATE MINDFULNESS INTO YOUR
DAILY ROUTINE TO SUPPORT YOUR TREATMENT?

Final Thoughts

THANK YOU FOR USING THIS JOURNAL AS A PART OF YOUR KETAMINE TREATMENT JOURNEY. REMEMBER, THIS IS A PERSONAL AND PRIVATE SPACE FOR YOUR REFLECTIONS. CONTINUE TO USE THESE PROMPTS AS NEEDED TO SUPPORT YOUR MENTAL HEALTH AND WELL-BEING.

GOOD LUCK ON YOUR JOURNEY!

Made in United States
Troutdale, OR
09/06/2024